Adrenal Reset Crash Course

Effective Diet & Exercise Solution for Adrenal Fatigue

By

Anne Peterson

SifuWilliam Lee

TABLE OF CONTENTS

Chapter 1 - Reasons of Weight Gain

- **Curb the calories**
- **Are carbohydrates your biggest enemy?**
- **Are you stuck with adrenal stress?**
- **Is exercise making you gain weight?**

Chapter 2 - The Role of Adrenal Glands in Weight Gain

- **Look for the warning signs**
- **Is your heart working right?**
- **Adrenal Gland Disorder**

Chapter3 - Final Debate on Proteins vs. Carbohydrates diet

- **Balanced diet**
- **Nutrition**
- **Intake**

Suggestions for Meals

- **Quinoa Salad (Serves 6)**
- **Vegetable Soup (Serves 6)**
- **Oatmeal Almond Delicacy (Serves 3)**
- **Protein shakes**
- **Energy soup**
- **Dinner Stir Fry**
- **Lunch Mixed Salad**

Chapter 9 - these foods are not limited in the Adrenal Reset Diet

Chapter 10 - Fruit

Chapter 11 – Qigong Exercise that Will Rejuvenate Your Life

Disclaimer

INTRODUCTION

This practical book is written so you can understand better what happens when your adrenal glands do not function properly. It has a main aim to simply explain reason why diets and exercise may not be working for you if your adrenal glands are not doing what they are designed to do. Most people already know if their hormones are not balanced, then their body does work properly. But they may not know exactly WHY hormones become unbalanced and WHAT one has to do in order to solve this deep-rooted problem of adrenal fatigue.

The purpose of this book is NOT only to help you understand the causes of the problem so many man and women face nowadays. One has to understand the nature of the problem in order to solve it but there is no need of studying these complex subject matters in debt. This guide is going to save your time but even better than that, it will help you to overcome this condition in smooth and easy way, by explaining everything, step by step.

Hormones are an essential part of our bodies. As you probably know they regulate our fat storage, our moods, emotions, metabolism, brain functions, and most importantly for some, our sex characteristics. When they do not work properly then the whole body suffers. Various other hormones are not produced and functions that are vital for the body to survive do not happen. The body needs to have its adrenal glands reset most probably, in order to go back to what it was.

Although the adrenal glands appear to be insignificant, they organize the rest of the body to a large extent. Found on top of both kidneys they seemingly are just lumps of spare tissue. But, without them, the human body would not produce insulin, vital for the metabolizing of sugar, male and female characteristics, the operations of the testes and the ovaries, and many functions that are more necessary.

Food comes under various guises, such as comfort, muscle building, brain food, cell-building and others, but often our diets do not help the adrenal glands to do their job and they grow tired. It is then that you may need to 'reset' them with a diet that actually feeds them and encourages them to go back to working, as they should.

Is This Book For You?

One of the first questions, which you have to answer, is "Are you reading the right book? "Many body problems can mimic others, so you need to be sure before embarking on a drastic change in your diet or exercise routine. You should also consult your doctor or health practitioner. I heavily recommend that you do this, and then come back to this book.

This book is written with the aim to help you and others who feel stressed out all the time without any reason. It may not be easy for you to look back and find out when the stress started setting in. It may also not be easy for you to make the needed changes in your lifestyle and give yourself a healthy and happy life. But once you start making the changes, you will feel the stress leaving your body automatically. Once you are into the phase of adrenal stress, you will need a lot of control over your body to get back to the normal routine. Though this is not an easy task, it is not a difficult one either. You have to make changes and ensure that you stick to the new routine.

As the adrenal glands become exhausted and cannot keep up with the body's demands, you will start seeing all the signs, which give you a clear indication that what you need is an Adrenal Reset Diet. This is one of the best means of getting back in shape. There are numerous recipes, which are included here; they are the stepping-stones to take you into a healthy lifestyle.

Once you commit to yourself to getting rid of this fatigue, all you need to do is follow the diet plan here. It will offer you simple means of changing your routine and give yourself much needed changes. If you are gaining weight at a faster pace, even though there is no change in your food intake routine, make sure that, you undergo the requisite tests to ensure that the functioning of your glands is under control. Your doctor can explain this further to you when he advises the appropriate tests to have.

In order to keep the hormones under control, you have to make sure that you avoid all such food items, which change the cortisol rhythm of your body. There are many dietary supplements, which offer you a balanced diet, which leads to improved health.

In the meantime

Here is a checklist, which may further provide you with an answer. If these symptoms are a part of your day-to-day life, you may be at the right place:

¨ **Feeling tired all the time.**
If you have had 8 hours good sleep, then you should not be still sleepy and tired when you wake. This is one of the most telling signs of Adrenal Gland Disorder. Sleep that does not involve nightmares or is disturbed is not a reason

to think you have Adrenal Disorder though.

¨ Small things stress you out

If you drop a cup on the floor and it shatters, this is not a life threatening disaster. If it sends you into hysterical bursts of tears though, it may show that you have Adrenal Stress. Of course, if the cup was very valuable, it may be a cause for misery, but still not hysterics.

¨ Fatigue right in the morning

Sleeplessness and broken sleep may make you tired and feeling irritable throughout the day. Usually you will get up with fatigue in the morning and feel lethargic or less willing to do the chores around the house. Your performance at work will be reduced and it may bring lot of disappointment and stress. A few people know their adrenal glands are behind all this trouble and their physical condition, and start to begin to fix the problem with small changes to their diet.

¨ Feeling lethargic and do not want to leave the bed in the morning.

You feel, as though you have run a marathon and your body just will not get its act together. In the end you roll over and try to go back to sleep. Seldom does this work and you spend the rest of your day alternately trying to work up the energy to get up or the energy to go back to sleep. Eventually you may force yourself to get up, only to be back in bed not an hour later.

¨ Feeling energetic (suddenly) in the evening time

You have slept all day, and did absolutely nothing, which did not concern you. Now, suddenly you spring to your fee and start attacking the washing, the washing up, tidying like a mad thing and your family stare at you in shock. This burst of energy naturally does not last long, and you are back on the bed again leaving everyone else in the household stunned and most of what you started undone.

¨ Mood swings

Mood swings are not only related to the pregnancy alone. You may have your mood changing faster than you were expecting when you are on some kind of medicine or treatment. A change in your adrenal glands is largely responsible for mood swings. Moods typically change several times a day, but sudden extreme mood swings are not proper, unless you are suffering from a diagnosed mental illness.

¨ Small things depress you

You look at a small amount of ironing that needs to be done. It may only be a shirt or a skirt, but the thought of having to iron it depresses you so much that you either leave it or wear something else instead. This is very common with Adrenals that need a reset in your diet.

¨ Get easily irritated

New parents and working moms often complain about such behaviors. Getting upset and irritated with children can lead to many complications that develop in their minds. For a busy worker or a mom, the first thing they should check out for is their adrenal gland working fine. In most cases, a little change in the diet and lifestyle can produce some great results and help them unwind and stay calm. If you find your Adrenals are not working as they should, it is easier to explain to your children that you have a condition that will change with attention. Involve them in making the meals and tell them that these will return you to the mother they knew.

¨ Nervousness

You have given the same talk for years. Now, you do not understand what you are talking about and think your listeners will be the same. You start to tense up and your words become spoken fast so you can get out of there. You do not encourage feedback or integration with your students or colleagues.

¨ Sugar cravings

When you wake up exhausted, your first point of call may be to make a cup of tea or coffee full of sugar. Or you may eat a bowl of some cereal loaded down with sugar to get your 'sugar fix'. Some even eat a full spoon of sugar straight down. This feeling of wanting sugar does not go away all through the day.

¨ Poor sleep

Do you toss and turn in bed all night long? Is there something that does not let you have some rest and you want to discuss with someone you trust? Or, is it just that you need to increase the adrenal levels in your body? Try that to get rid of poor sleep disorder by changing your diet but without the need of heavy pills or any other way of treatment.

¨ Decreasing sex drive

Did you know your adrenal glands not working properly are responsible for your loss of desire and less libido? Hormones, which control these feelings, are in turn controlled by the release of hormones from the adrenal glands. Start using natural energy filled shakes and drinks to increase the working of adrenal glands in your body and enhance your sex drive.

¨ Hands and feet get cold all the time (or to often)

As we age, our hands and feet feel cold due to circulatory problems in many cases. But when your Adrenals need a reset, those extremities of our bodies feel frozen and do not warm up. The circulation is fine; as are the nerve endings, but our hands and feet still feel frozen. Resetting your Adrenal Glands by changing your diet will help this uncomfortable feeling go away.

¨ Excessive weight gain

Did you have sudden increase in your weight? It may be the lack of nutrition, obsessive eating disorder or it can be just your adrenals. Many people join gyms and spend a great deal of money on sporting gear, but it may not do you any good if your adrenals are not in good shape. Try fixing your diet to help the adrenals before splashing out on expensive gym memberships and equipment.

¨ Joint pain

Your joints may be painful to flex or move with no obvious reason. Especially if you have no history of early onset of arthritis in your family or other joint diseases. The adrenal glands regulate the amount of lubrication that is distributed in and around the joints when they are in action, thus keeping them easily moving.

¨ Intolerance towards heat

Most people feel uncomfortable after a while if they sit too close to a radiator. This is natural. However, if it is a beautiful day that is not too hot or warm and you dislike being out in it because you feel very hot and you are not wearing a jacket or warm clothing, then you may need an Adrenal Reset Diet.

¨ Salty food cravings

A lot of people have the craving for salty foods. If you cannot resist and keep your hands off salted nuts, crackers and biscuits, you are just lacking something in your adrenal diet. It is one of the major signs of adrenal glands not providing adequate amounts of necessary hormones in your body.

Have you ticked any of or a lot of these points? You really should get yourself checked out either by your health practitioner or your doctor and have some blood samples taken for tests for adrenal functioning. If you are a young healthy person or simply think you are healthy, then any or all of these symptoms may show you to be suffering from needing an Adrenal Reset Diet. The Adrenal Glands dysfunctions may not be noticed for some time down the track, so it is important you keep an eye on whether these symptoms grow quickly, the same as you would with a strange mole that suddenly appears.

If you are experiencing one, some or many of these symptoms, make sure that you go through this book. This is one book, which will provide you with complete information on how to handle stress and lead a normal lifestyle, but it is not a substitute for your health practitioner or your doctor.

Make a checklist of the symptoms listed above and then find out how many of them relate to you. If your list is comprehensive, you need to start taking steps towards improving your adrenal health and leading a healthy life in the future. Check with your doctor or health practitioner and begin a healthy diet change.

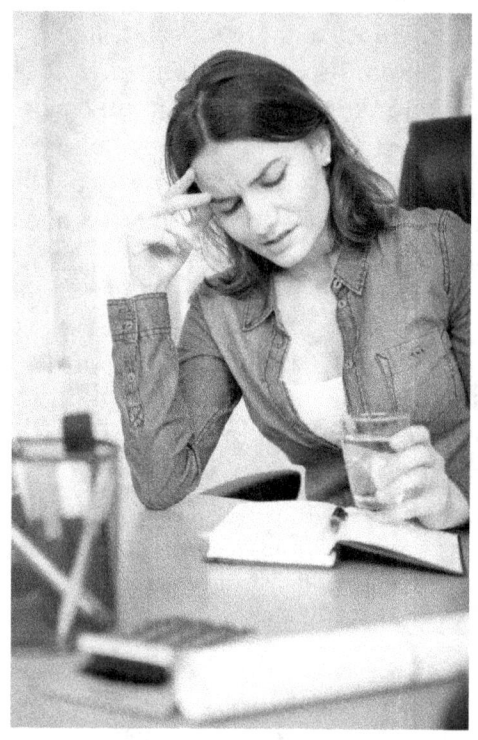

Why Listen To Us?

We will give you very short and clear answer. We know this type of collaboration is not seen often however since we have received fantastic positive response on Happy & Gluten Free - Lifestyle Guide book, we decided to publish this guide as well. Readers that have found useful our Gluten Free Lifestyle Guide are not necessarily in need of Adrenal Reset practice and vice versa. However, these conditions are sort of connected and we deal with them practically on daily basis.

About Anne Peterson

"In answer to the above question, ("why listen to these authors...") there are quite few reasons you could find strong and valid. There is probably one reason that dominates all others. Few decades of Veganism and consulting experience are great but having two children; both suffering from two different forms of sensitivity to Gluten does make a difference. On top of that during mid 80's not many people (including the medical personal) knew much about hypersensitivity to Gluten and related conditions, right? Long story short, being affectionate and loving mother dedicated to understand the matter and find the best way to help their children makes Anne 'authority' in this field. Not a doctor, not a professor but real and authentic expert.

I am very happy we have met on time. Accepting any client, especially young mother with two kinds, boy and the girl that suffer is a challenge. I am so pleased I have accepted that challenge and despite of the complexity, I did not turned away from that chance. I have learned many things due to our relationship that grew over the years. One of the amazing discoveries I got to is how modern alternative approach is not at all distant from the views of Traditional Chinese Medicine if you just know how to compare them".

Written by Sifu William Lee, 2nd March 2015, Zhengzhou, China

About Sifu William Lee

"It is very difficult for me to fit answer on this question in just few lines. Sifu Lee is just personification of advanced science and practices related to TCM (Traditional Chinese Medicine) that aren't at all simple to understand and yet he is teaching everything in a way that is so easy to understand and apply. Everyone familiar with his books knows that and no one of his readers or students need any introduction. I have enormous amount of respect and gratefulness towards him and his work – without his help I would experience a lot longer way to solutions I had to find for my family. In this world, people like Sifu Lee are extremely rare gems.

Now, if you do not know much about him, let me share you one thing with you. His approach to anything, as well as to matters of healing and health is hitting the root cause of the problems. He is not wasting any time and energy with theoretical explanations and such but is dealing with the very cause of a problem – that is fantastic! And one more thing – you know that Chinese proverb "If you want to help to hungry man do not feed him but teach him to fish..." THAT exactly is what Sifu Lee is all about and I have no words to express my gratefulness for everything he did and for willing to co author this book with me."

Adrenal Reset Diet Crash Course

*Written by Anne Peterson, 4th
March 2015, Fairfield, Iowa, US*

Why This Book?

Using just few words, answer would be "in order to help you avoid mistakes and save (a lot of) your time, energy and MONEY!" You probably already have your own experience – things that are complicated, normally are not effective and are simply just too demanding. Just like aperson suffering from gluten intolerance,you as well have too many choices – there are so many diet plans, cookbooks, information ... that may sometimes be really confusing. Yes, fact is that man and women affected with celiac disease are not alone. Different support groups are active in giving support and there are other sides that offer the support yet it is very important to know *whom to listen and who better not – similarly there are those from whom advice we better stay away.*

In this book therefore, you can get all the information related to adrenal reset diet and alternative support to refreshing the adrenal glad functioning.

Healthy functioning of our body, internal organs and all systems within our bodies are dependent to flow of energy - adrenal gland and related health issues are directly influenced and first to suffer when a Qi flow (flow of life energy) is disturbed.

This effective recovery method you are getting in this chapter, you can't easily find elsewhere – ancient meridian stretching exercises presented by Sifu William Lee, a known author of many great books about healing, Qigong, acupressure and related themes. Because ofhis expert insight, ancient methods of Traditional Chinese Medicine are presented here in order to guarantee efficiency and simplicity.

Now just few more words about unique thing are that you just can't find elsewhere. In our guide, you will find simple yet powerful routine, presented in Amazon bestselling books authored by Sifu William Lee. Book Total Chi Fitness is explaining these methods in details, yet here we will offer you basic idea followed by a Free Video.

These ancient Chinese methods are extremely potent and will diminish your symptoms by 20-30% in first few weeks!

And anyone will agree, the best is that anyone can add these methods in to daily routine without much trouble and pain sinceit can take only12 -15 minutes of time. About that, we will give you all details in later chapters - this ancient Qigong routine we present in book will simply surprise you, by its simplicity and powerful potency.

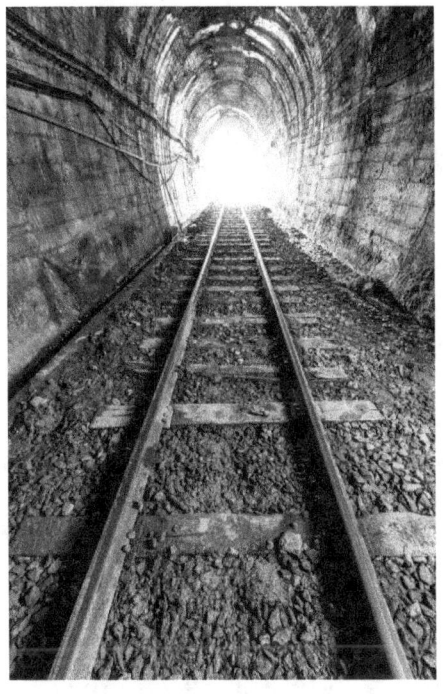

Who May Need An Adrenal Reset Diet?

The incidence of obesity is growing ever more common across the world, despite the proliferation of gyms and diets. Even countries, which are considered poor, are becoming fat. And there does not seem to be one consistent reason for this. Diets of fast food, little exercise, lack of fresh food in the diet, the amount of pesticides and chemicals used to grow food, the list of perhaps causes is endless, but there also seems to be very little in the way to stop this avalanche of fat people.

People are also becoming larger through genetic changes. But there is still no obvious reason why even very young people seem to be becoming fat at an early stage of life. True, many people seem to eat only heavily processed foods, but also many of them do not gain weight rapidly. They appear to have energy to burn and you can only sit back and envy them.

Some people can eat anything they like and not gain an ounce. I am not disbelieving this for one minute. People with healthy Adrenal Glands have optimum levels of hormones dealing with simple or complex stress and may not exercise overly but seem to handle every challenge with grace and equanimity. Wouldn't you like to be like them? Then just reset your Adrenal Glands through your diet.

This is just generalizing, of course, but this fact is still there. Many people suffer from hormonal problems and the Adrenals are two of the most important hormone producing tissues in the body. Furthermore, they regulate other hormone producing tissues as well, so it makes sense if the adrenals are not working properly then the rest of the hormone producing organs are not either.

Not everyone will need to reset his or her adrenal glands through diet. But those who have tried all of the channels to lose weight and find themselves not doing so should ideally have themselves checked over properly by a doctor, have themselves tested for how their adrenals are working or not, and then, will the doctor's permission, commence a trial of the Adrenal Reset Diet.

There are drugs, which cause us to gain weight. Unfortunately, these drugs are often those, which help our bodies regulate other things, such as high blood pressure, diabetes, etc. This is why it is so important for you to get your doctor's approval before you start any diet, including this one.

The Basic Concept Of Adrenal Reset Diet

Carbs eaten early in the morning are thought to settle as fat around the middle of the body, although the fat may settle anywhere. The concept of this diet is that the later in the day carbs are consumed the better because it allows them less time to settle. Of course, the least amount of carbs you can consume the better, which is why this diet uses little or few carbs and mostly vegetables.

These contain fiber, minerals and vitamins, but no carbs. Unlike some types of soup, you can use the ones here for breakfast should you wish. Soup is a filling meal and the one mentioned here is good whether it be for breakfast or your last meal of the day.

There are not many breads involved in this diet, nor any heavy carbohydrates. If you wish soup to have bread with it, it is recommended you use less liquid to make the soup so it is thicker. Most breadis thick with carbohydrates. Add grains from the list provided. Dairy milk is used in moderation.

Reasons To Think Of Adopting An Adrenal Reset Diet

Are you feeling tired and fatigued for no reason at all? Do you feel stressed out for no particular reason? There are many stress related symptoms, which you should take into count. Do you have outside pressures that may be contributing to your feelings of misery? Take steps if possible to counter these and see if you feel any better. If not, then dig deeper into this eBook.

Continuous experience of stress and trauma should be warning signs for you. If you are unable to leave your bed in the morning, there are chances that you are suffering from Adrenal Fatigue Syndrome. Some of the most obvious symptoms which you can easily see and feel are fatigue, insomnia, cannot get up in the morning and then there is a sudden burst of energy in the afternoon or evening.

When your adrenal glands, pituitary gland and hypothalamus do not function up to the optimum level, you are bound to suffer from this condition. The adrenal glands play a pivotal role in the overall function of your body. They have control over the vital organs and ensure that your body functions in a normal manner. One of the most important roles, which are played by this gland, is to ensure that the stress releasing hormones like DHEA, cortisol, epinephrine, etc. have control over your body's response. These hormones are important for regulating your heart rate, enhancing your immune system, normalizing your energy storage and ensuring the overall functionality of your body.

The chief function of these hormones is to control stress related symptoms and ensure that they function at the optimum level. Now you must be wondering what is Adrenal Reset Diet? The basic concept is to make changes in your diet pattern in such a way so that the adrenal glands function in a normal manner. Once you start on this diet, you will immediately see the change in the way you feel. Getting out of bed early in the morning will no longer be a stressful exercise for you. No longer will you feel tired even after a long sleep.

Adrenal Reset Diet – Myth Vs. Reality

Once you know that you are suffering from adrenal fatigue, you have to start looking for ways to get away from stress. There are many theories floating around which throw away the concept of adrenal reset diet and the best means of removing stress related to adrenal gland disorder. Taking charge of your diet is perhaps the best way to help your adrenal glands work efficiently once again.

We firmly believe that if you make sufficient change in your diet, you are able to take control over your adrenal glands and be set to lead a healthy life. Before we embark on the need of this diet, let us clear some of the myths, which are the foundation of this diet program. Below are the 3 biggest myths of adrenal tiredness:

1.   Adrenal Gland Fatigue

Are you gaining weight on a continuous basis, no matter what you do or eat? If this is the case, there are chances that you are suffering from adrenal fatigue. What is the adrenal gland? They are tiny lumps of tissue, which are found right on top of our kidneys. There are numerous hormones produced by these glands, which are important in the normal function of your body. These hormones play a pivotal role in controlling the energy level of your body, your weight and the way you respond to stress.

But conventional doctors are not in support of this concept. According to them, these glands do not get tired, lose their efficiency and cause these symptoms. This debate has been on for a long time. If your adrenal glands malfunction, there are strong chances that you get autoimmune disorders, which would affect your entire lifestyle to name one of the problems, which indicate your adrenals are not functioning properly.
If you get stressed a lot, there are chances of you getting heart disease, lack

of sleep, obesity and anxiety. A lot of stress is harmful for your adrenal, and would mean that there is a loss of the delicate balance that the body needs.

The reality is that the adrenal gland, like other parts of the body, does have a tiredness level. There are several glands of which the adrenal glands are a part and the entire cluster is called the Hypothalamic Pituitary Adrenal (HPA) axis. A disorder of this set of glands might lead to adrenal stress. Once these glands start functioning normally, there will be sufficient cortisol generated in the body to ensure normal operation of your body.

2.   You Need A Lot Of Medication For Your Adrenal

When your adrenal glands do not function in the proper manner, it means that your body is not making the right amount of cortisol. This means you have to take medication in order to balance its level in your body. Whenever there is an imbalance in your body, you have to take corrective steps in order to ensure its proper functioning. There are many different herbs and pills, which will assist you in improving your cortisol level. Ensure you consult a doctor or a qualified person before you go self-medicating yourself so you can be sure of being on the right track.

But if you wish to avoid medication, there are also many other natural means by which you can change your cortisol level. One of the best ways to do this is to sit out in the open under the sunlight. This should be done after you wake up in the morning. Without wearing sunglasses, sit in the open within an hour after you wake up. If this exercise is done on a regular basis, you are sure to see marked change in your cortisol level within a very short period of time.

Use low voltage bulbs of red color in your bedroom. When you are sitting in your bedroom at night, reading a book, make sure that you use this light for the process. Close all the doors and windows, block all the passages of light and use this red colored light only in the evenings and nighttime. It is not advised you read for too long though. Variants of 10 - 30 minutes are usually quite long enough.

These natural means will help give you freedom from pills and will give you much needed freedom from some type of medication therapy. However, you still need your doctor or health worker to keep a professional eye on what your adrenals are doing.

3.   Once adrenal stress sets in, you cannot get rid of it

Is adrenal stress chronic? Is there nothing you can do to get rid of it? Well this myth is dismissed. There are many simple means by which you can get rid of adrenal stress. One of the best ways is to make changes in your diet; add food, which is good for you, and get rid of such foods, which enhance your stress level. A change in your diet plan will take you a long way in changing your body and how it is functioning.

There is not much you have to do. You just have to moderate your diet a little. Just making changes and taking in food, which is good for you, and avoiding food, which will harm you, will do the trick. You will feel a complete change in the way your body reacts and will feel a lot more energetic.

Chapter 1

REASONS OF WEIGHT GAIN

Stress plays a vital role in the hormonal changes of your body. This leads to breaking down of tissues and major change in the hormonal balance. There are many diseases like diabetes, heart related diseases, obesity, autoimmune diseases, rheumatoid arthritis, hypothyroidism, and other hormonal related diseases, which are affected by your stress management. Stress in moderation is good, because it encourages organs to work efficiently. However, like everything, too much stress over a long period of time will damage the body.

With hormonal imbalance, come many other disorders of which the most important one is obesity. No matter what you eat and how much you eat, if your adrenal glands are not working efficiently and producing the hormones the liver needs, you are sure to convert it into fat, which is stored in your body. This increases your weight dramatically and also leads to mood swings. The most affected system of your body is your metabolism. This means that the food, which should be otherwise utilized, is converted into fats and stored in your body, leading to excessive weight gain.

1.   Curb the calories?

Will it really work? Can you control your calorie intake and lose weight, which you have, adrenal fatigue? The answer to this question is most likely no. The major reason behind the fact you cannot lose weight is that the hormonal imbalance which is a part of your body now. What you need to do first is to ensure that you get the hormones back under your control.

Are you eating food, which is high in carbohydrates? If the answer to this question is yes, you need to make major changes in the diet and remove them from your food. Carbohydrates are your biggest enemy after stress and will not allow your body to adapt to the much-needed change.

2. Are carbohydrates your biggest enemy?

The answer is yes; not because carbohydrates in it are harmful, but because there is no proper utilization of carbohydrates in the body. Carbohydrates, when absorbed naturally by the body, are one of the biggest sources of energy. But you have to understand that your body is different. It is no longer ready or capable of digesting carbohydrates and this could be the reason why you see so many obese people in the streets these days. Of course, not all of them will have problems with their adrenal glands but the possibility is high.

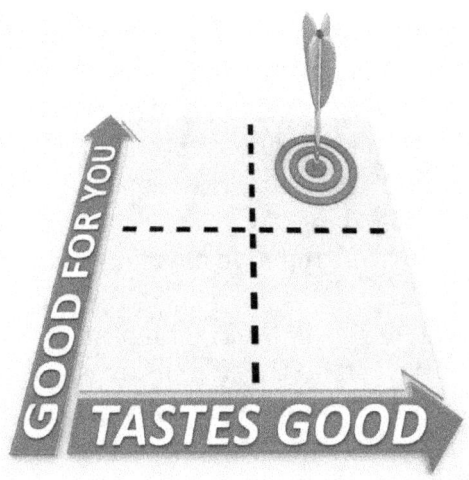

If you take the right amount of carbohydrates, in a form, which is digestible, you will be able to get the best out of the food, which you consume. If you handle stress in a better manner, you will also be able to absorb carbs. Though a difficult proposition, it is not an impossible one. You have to give your body time and also ensure that you are using a healthy food chart.

3. Are you weighed down with adrenal stress?

One of the most common symptoms of adrenal fatigue is to feel lethargic the time. A sudden burst of energy, which is the fight or flight reaction to a perceived real or unreal danger can be very dangerous to the heart if it is continual. This one symptom is the most dangerous. The reason being that you aretrapped in a vicious cycle. Your body does not process carbohydrates in the right manner anymore and on top of that, stress is killing you. Once you are stuck with this symptom, you are going to have a hard time in getting rid of it. However, it is not impossible. You just have to make some important dietary changes.

Adrenal stress affects the moods of your body, and this is one of the most important functions of all. People do not like dealing with someone whom they cannot trust to be in one mood one minute, only to become Mr. Hyde the next. Not only is it stressful for the person involved, it is also very stressful for the sufferer. A metabolism malfunction would lead to mood swings and many other things that offer to enhance stress levels. Every little or big thing becomes a disaster of heroic proportions.

4. Is exercise making you fat?

Many of us know that sinking feeling of when you have almost killed yourself at the gym or some other way of exercising and the weight continues to creep on. It is depressing, infuriating and most of all, very encouraging of despair, especially if you are stressing yourself out trying to find the energy to continue to exercise. There is another source of stress right there on your doorstep and you don't realize it.

Exercise is one of the important factors that allow us to function in wellness. But exercise may also make us feel sick, tired and depressed if our adrenal glands are not working to optimum standards. The Adrenal Reset Diet will help to return exercise to something to be enjoyed not endured, as well as aiding it in getting rid of the weight which is mysteriously still growing.

Natural foods feed the muscles so they can function as they were intended to do. If the muscles cannot access the proper needs for them, they are likely to react in unexpected ways. Bones also become, over a period of time, brittle as they are not subjected to exercise and fed foods, which do not strengthen them. In processed foods diets, the process of refining removes many of the necessary minerals for bone strength.

CHAPTER 2

THE ROLE OF ADRENAL GLANDS IN WEIGHT GAIN

The adrenal glands are two very small essential lumps of tissue, which are located above each of your kidneys. Though small in size, they have major responsibilities. The most important functions of these glands are to secrete hormones, which balance the overall functioning of your body. Some of the chemicals produced are Cortisol, DHEA, adrenal, aldosterone, etc. When these glands are working at their optimum the body receives what hormones it needs at the right times, such as feelings of stress, hunger, etc. When the hormones are not released when they are needed, several bad changes begin to happen.

Emotions become very hard to predict, even for the sufferer. Some people are capable of foreseeing an attack of an emotion out of control but many are not. Not only does this add to the stress of the situation, but also it often leads to deep and very dark depression whereby the person suffering will not go out in public for fear of the emotions that may spring free. Weight gain is often the least of their problems, because they do not trust themselves around others. On the other hand others do not like being around them, so they suffer in two ways.

If these necessary hormones are not in controlled release, you are likely to be showing signs of fatigue. For example, if proper cortisol level is not maintained, you are sure to see growth in your tummy region within no time. Similarly, there will be fat deposits all over your body. When the body is unable to convert carbohydrates and fats into energy, you are bound to suffer from general fatigue. The hormones secreted by the adrenal glands control all this. This is the reason why these glands play a major role in weight gain.

1. Look for the warning signs

If you start feeling that maybe adrenal fatigue has started setting in, it is time for you tobegin looking for the warning signs. One of the major signs is weight gain and the inability to lose it. If this is the case, make sure that you make the right changes to your diet and cut off one of the culprit's right at the root.

If you are feeling restless and tired for no reason at all, you should start thinking of trying the Adrenal reset diet and see if this brings your body back somewhere to normal before things get out of hand. Some of the typical signs of needing an Adrenal Reset Change to your diet include:

- Suffering lack of sleep at night and feeling lethargic during the daytime.
- Not wanting to leave the bed in the morning and
- For the entire day, you feel very sluggish and lazy.
- Come 6pm or onwards for a short time, you will feel a sudden gust of energy and want to finish all the work immediately.

- Salt and sugar cravings are another set of symptoms of adrenal fatigue.
- Also, you will not be able to maintain proper health all the time.
- As your immune system will be down, you will get one or another infection and you will remain ill for longer than the normal span of the illness.

These are some of the most common warning symptoms, which you should pay, heed to.

2. Is your heart working right?

The change in hormones also tends to affect the functioning of your heart. If you feel slightest chest pain or discomfort, make sure that you immediately consult a doctor. Once you have adrenal fatigue, it is imperative that you keep getting the condition of your heart checked time and again. Malfunctioning adrenal glands place strain on a lot of body parts, which you may not comprehend. Anyslightest problem in the chest area should not be ignored and proper attention to it should be paid.

3. Adrenal Gland Disorder

When the adrenal glands are not working properly, many disorders occur. The body starts to be lazy, wants no exercise and craves salt or sugar or sometimes both. Below are listed a few of the serious problems that can occur when the adrenal glands are not working:

- Craving salty foods. An excess of salt in the kidneys increases the amount of water that it keeps back, which in turn often leads to the blood pressure being pushed up into dangerous levels. The kidneys do not do so well when they are loaded with salt and so start to be damaged.

- The body cannot exist in a continual cycle of flight or fight mode. This is exhausting for the heart and the lungs.
- The immune system becomes weakened, leading to frequent infections such as continually having the flu or viruses staying far longer than their cycle is.

- Weight gain is fast and will not go away, even when diets and exercise are applied.

- Hormone changes occur. The adrenal glands are responsible for creating the male and female hormones. Females may find themselves developing male characteristics while males may find the same happening of the opposite type. Females may begin to find hair growing on their chests and elsewhere abnormal while males may find their testes beginning to shrink. Mood swings can be violent and sudden.

- One of the purposes of the adrenal glands is to produce glucocorticoids, which help the liver produce glucose. When this important function is disrupted, the body experiences potential life threatening problems.

- The production of cortisol. Without this substance, your body will not function at all well and the lack of it is life threatening.

- Healthy food is not appealing.

So, as you can see, adrenal gland disorder leads to many other disorders and dysfunctions of your body. Gaining weight rapidly, fast unexplained changes in mood, a very low sex drive, exhaustion, change in metabolism, etc. are some of the most important symptoms of adrenal gland disorder.

Feeling tired and lazy keeps you away from exercise and also offers you excuses having a poor diet. The laziness in you grows beyond bounds and all this combined leads to a very stressful situation. This affects and disrupts your life and forces you to lead a life full of

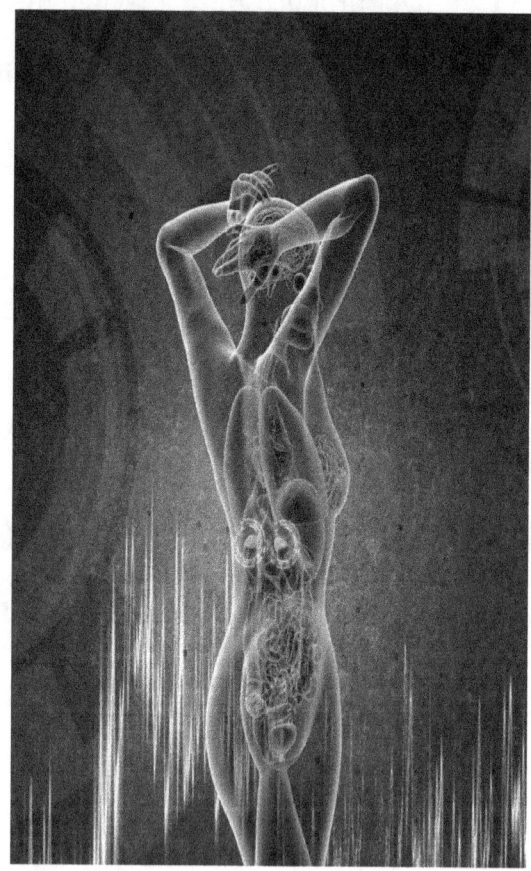

laziness and stress. Usually both at the same time.

Chapter 3

Final Debate On Proteins Vs. Carbohydrates Diet

A balanced diet is what you are looking for here to control adrenaline and lead a stress free life. Yes, you can make the changes needed in your lifestyle to ensure a healthy life. What is required is a change in diet and restoration of the proper adrenal function,

Proteins are important to give your body the required controlled release of energy and help with the building of new cells. Carbohydrates, on the other hand can turn out to be your enemy if you do not take them in a controlled manner. Both proteins and carbohydrates are necessary for the body to function, but a diet of pure carbohydrates or one of proteins is not good. When you eat one or the other solely, you miss out on what is needed from the other. With an adrenal reset diet, the balance between the two is restored and allows both nutrients to be used.

1. Balanced diet

What you are looking for here is a balanced diet, which would provide you with a balanced lifestyle. Once you have control over your food intake, you will be able to get control over the glands, which cause stress in your life and get motivated to improve your exercise pattern. Giving the body the required amount of food of the required quality is the master key to a healthy life.

Once the adrenal glands are back to their normal selves, you will start losing weight, feel energetic, attain self-control, and will start feeling alive again. This may seem a hard task that is perhaps handled with medications, but it can be done with the right mix of nutrition. Nutrition can help the tablets out enormously if you opt for taking tablets instead.

2. Nutrition

In a race to attain proper health, make sure that you do not lose out on the nutrition part. Though there are some food items, which are poison to your body, make sure that you take proper supplements to maintain the balance. You may be advised by your doctor to take certain supplements if you cannot get enough of them in your diet. However gaining them through what you eat is far better than artificially consuming them.

Proper food, prepared in the right manner, is the trigger, which will take you towards a healthy lifestyle. Just make sure that you take food with the right amount of nutritional value and this is the first step towards a healthy life. Not all food is right for fixing the adrenal gland, but you can learn what is by finishing reading this eBook.

3. Intake

What you are eating is more important here rather than how much you are eating. The entire diet should be planned in such a manner that you have the right amount of control over calories and at the same time get the proper nutrition. A balanced diet is an ideal intake for you to get rid of the adrenal fatigue. Once the adrenal glands start functioning in normal manner, there would be no need for you to follow such strict regime.

Chapter 4

The Importance Of Adrenal Reset Diet In Your Life

Adrenal fatigue leads to many problems, which affect your physical and mental health. With the onset of symptoms of adrenal fatigue, it is important that you start taking proper steps to get back into shape both mentally and physically.

Once depression sets in, it becomes difficult for you to recover fast. Slowly and steadily, laziness would creep in and you would be completely lost. This is when you should adopt the adrenal reset diet. Depression is very bad for anyone and should not be allowed to develop.

Get in shape

In order to get back in shape, what you require the most is to get the reins of your life in your hands. Make the required changes in your diet in order to get back in shape. With increasing stress levels, you might find it difficult to respond to the measures having to be taken to reduce stress. But with determination and persistence, you are sure to neutralize stress and lead a healthy life once again.

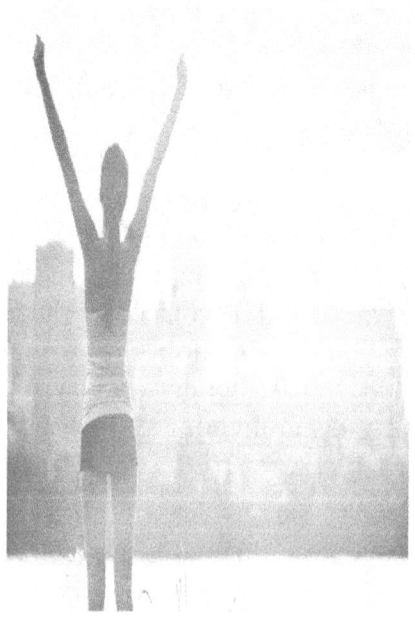

CHAPTER 5

KNOW WHERE YOU STAND

Before you go off in a rush to change everything you are doing, get your doctor to perform all the relevant tests and discuss the possibility of you needing an adrenal diet reset. It is most important to get the right diagnosis made before embarking on this program. You do not want to find that your symptoms stay around even when you have changed your diet and done everything else correctly, only to find you have been treating the wrong thing.

Not that this can be a bad mistake, but it is always better to be safe than sorry. Sometimes trying to treat a condition, which is not confirmed, may make a positive change to your body anyway, but it can also hide something else away which is not good.

So again, I urge you to follow the below instructions and be sure of what you are trying to fix.

1. **What to do:**

Make a proper assessment of your health. Undergo proper tests to find out your sugar levels, the condition of your heart, cortisol levels in your body and other tests, which are suggested by your doctor. This will tell you where you stand as far as your physical health are concerned. Once you have the results in your hand, you will know the exact state of your body and this should be the trigger to make the required changes in your lifestyle.

2. **Control the stress**

One of the most important things, which you have to do, is get an upper hand on the stress. There will be many instances in your life where you will feel stressed out for a reason or for no reason at all. When you reach a stage, where there is so much stress in life that it brings in negativity, sickness, tiredness and depression sets in within no time, you need to find a cure, fast. And starting organizing or reorganizing your diet should be your first move back towards health.

When you hear the first warning bell, it is time for you to take the reins of your life in your hands. Controlling stress is the first step towards leading a healthy life.

It is normal for a body to react to stress and enhance the levels of cortisol in the body. The body has a fight or flight pattern that has come through from the time when one wrong move meant probably being eaten. This might lead to infection and inflammation nowadays. Heartburn, gas, bloating, etc. are some of the common signs of this disorder. In women, there are many hormonal disorders, which are related to adrenal fatigue. Some of the most common include irregular menstrual cycle, infertility, etc.

3. Check your Adrenal levels

Modern day technology has improved and progressed and now

provides complete and accurate information which will give you a clear picture of the state of health of your body. With the correct tests, you can determine the exact cause of adrenal insufficiency. This diagnosis detects the adrenal levels and will provide you with the clear understanding of the reasons of adrenal fatigue.

The three main organs of our body, which play a role in adrenal fatigue, are the hypothalamus, the adrenal gland and the pituitary gland. Ensure that these three are functioning in the proper manner and you will get this stress back under control within no time. The hormones, which are secreted by these glands, are responsible for the enhanced level of stress. Proper levels are whatare required to lead a healthy life.

4. **Mainstream medicine vs. change in diet**

There are many medications, which are available in the market, which will offer you relief from the stress and at the same time balance, your hormones.

But the temporary change, which is brought about by this medication, is reversible and within no time, you will start observing the symptoms again.

One of the best ways to bring a turnabout is to change your diet and make sure that you do not take in any food, which affects the functioning of these glands. Set a program for yourself and follow it strictly. This will give you the much-needed energy for a healthy and happy life.

CHAPTER 6

THE GIST OF ADRENAL RESET DIET – A HEALTHY LIFE

Changing lifestyle and proper diet are the stepping-stones towards a healthy life. Getting a release from stressful lives is a dream comes true for many people. Though this is a stage, which is not easy to achieve, you can reach there with strict control over your own body and what you put in it in the way of food.

Changing your diet and eating the right meals at the right time will give you a healthy mind and a fit body. A healthy body and mind is what many people crave all the time and is difficult to achieve. But if by starting to make changes in eating habits, you will restore your original health is enough motivation to start healing yourself then why not go for it?

CHAPTER 7

RESET THE ADRENAL DIET

There are steps, which will give you back the right health and relieve all the stress and stain from your body. Some of the most affected areas of the body are mood, immune system and metabolism. With the proper intake of food, you can easily manage these three areas and get a healthy body as a bonus.

Of course, you will need to experiment to see what combinations of vegetables suit you best. However, there are so many vegetables involved that you should never get bored. So, follow the below tips and tasty suggestions for meals and start your way back to health!

a) Check with your doctor to find out whether an Adrenal Reset Diet is going to help you. Being a diet that includes a lot of vegetables and little carbohydrates it may not be suitable for you. Carbohydrates are not all evil and the body does need some for optimum function. Perhaps you can modify the Diet to include some carbs, or practice it for short periods of time. Once you have the Adrenals back under control, it is not necessary to continue to be so strict with your diet.

b) Take some exercise. If you were training hard, ease up on that until you feel the benefits of the Adrenal Reset Diet kicking in, then up your exercise quota until you are back where you were before.

c) Keep taking your medications. This is very important. The Diet will work with them to optimize their effects but it is only on your doctor's say-so that you should ever cease taking medications.

The Adrenal Reset Diet is not a quick cure-all, but it is one, which, over a period of time, will regulate your Adrenal Glands back to normal. You will notice a change in your moods for the better, your body will lose that sluggish feeling and you will have energy again.

CHAPTER 8.

BUILD YOUR HEALTH WITH HEALTHY DIET

You will notice that quinoa is used regularly in this diet as an aid to restore the adrenal glands to order. This is because this grain has long been known to have health giving properties. For thousands of years it has been a staple of diets that are very low in carbohydrates, yet have high values of health.

Quinoa is fairly easily digested, has more filling properties than rice, corn or other grains and has less potential for bloating, which is also a part of some other grains. It can be used in soups, shakes or smoothies and other main meals to impart a more filling feeling to them.

The list of unlimited vegetables has been chosen for the different properties that the vegetables hold. Few of them have starch, another reason for causes of bloat and all have fiber, good for bowel health. Each vegetable also has other benefits for such various organs such as eyes and the heart.

Suggestions For Meals

Examples of meals used in the Adrenal Reset Diet.

Quinoa Salad (Serves 6)

One of the most popular grains to control adrenal fatigue is Quinoa. It is a balanced grain, the chief ingredient of which is thiamine, zinc, copper, vitamin B6, riboflavin, dietary fiber, etc. This recipe is quick to make and will quench your food craving very efficiently.

Ingredients:
1. 1 cup of dry quinoa
2. 1/2 cup finely chopped parsley

3.   1/4 cup chopped cucumber
4.   1/4 cup chopped coriander
5.   1/4 cup fresh chickpeas
6.   1/4 cup chopped mint leaves
7.   2 medium tomatoes finely chopped
8.   4 tablespoons olive oil
9.   1 teaspoon lemon juice
10. Salt, jalapenos' and pepper to taste

How to make

1. Boil 2 cups of water.
2. Add quinoa and keep stirring for 20 minutes or until cooked.
3. Once cooked, use the fork to fluff the quinoa and keep aside to cool.
4. Mix all the other ingredients in a separate bowl.
5. Once the quinoa is cool, add the other ingredients and serve garnished with coriander leaves.
6. You can also garnish with finely chopped onion.

Vegetable Soup (Serves 6)

This is a recipe, which takes longer to cook as it has to be done slowly in order to get the right flavor. Make sure that you have enough patience to make this one! This soup contains all the vital ingredients needed to get your adrenal working and in order.

Ingredients
a) 4c water
b) 1 finely chopped onion
c) 1 tablespoon fresh garlic chopped finely
d) 6 finely chopped tomatoes
e) 1 large sliced zucchini
f) 1 cup chickpeas
g) 2 sliced carrots
h) 1 bay leaf
i) Salt and pepper to taste

How to make

a) Once the water starts boiling, add bay leaf, garlic, onion, garlic and salt and pepper.
b) Keep boiling at a low flame.

c) Keep this pot on the flame for 3-4 hours.
d) Add the chopped vegetables and other ingredients to the pot.
e) Bring it again to boil and simmer for about 15 minutes or until the vegetables become soft.
f) Serve hot, garnished with coriander leaves. You can also add a few drops of lemon to add the tinge.

Oatmeal Almond Delicacy (Serves 3)

Ingredients

1. 1/4 cup oats, preferable gluten-free
2. 1/2 cup unsweetened almond milk
3. 2/3 cup natural almond butter
4. Vanilla pea protein powder, 1 serving

How to make

1. Mix almond butter and milk in a microwave safe glass bowl.
2. Place in the microwave for approximately 2 minutes or till the butter turns soft.
3. Take the bowl from the microwave and mix the butter and milk.
4. Once the batter is smooth, stir in the protein powder.
5. Make sure that there are no lumps and that powder completely blends in the milk butter combination.
6. Once this is done, add the gluten-free oats and stir.
7. Once the entire batter is ready, make small rolls and put in the refrigerator for 20 minutes.
8. Serve once the tasty rolls are hard.

Protein shakes

Ingredients

1. 1 Frozen banana
2. 2 tablespoons protein powder
3. 2 tablespoon green powder

4. Half frozen avocado
5. 4 tablespoons frozen blueberries
6. 3 tablespoon plain yogurt
7. 1 tablespoon coconut oil
8. 1 cup soy milk
9. Salt to taste
10. Water as needed

How to make

1. Mix all ingredients in the blender and blend smooth.
2. Mix ice cubes if you want a cooler version.
3. This is a health drink, which will give you instant energy.
4. Each ingredient has its own nutritional value and will give your day a healthy start.

Energy soup

Ingredients

1. 1/2 onion, finely chopped
2. 2 carrots, finely chopped
3. 1 cup chickpeas
4. 1 cup finely chopped broccoli

5. 3 garlic cloves, chopped
6. 3 diced celery stalks
7. Salt and lemon to taste
8. 2 tablespoon olive oil

How to make

1. Heat the oil and add garlic, celery, onion and carrots.
2. Cook over medium heat for around 7 minutes, or until tender.
3. Add chickpeas and broccoli and again cook at medium heat for about 2 minutes.
4. Add 4 cups of water and let it simmer until the vegetables turn tender.
5. Switch off the gas and let it cool for some time.
6. Add salt and lemon and serve.

Dinner Stir Fry

Ingredients

1. 1 cup of soybean
2. Take a selection of vegetables from the list provided below

3. Use soy sauce, ginger, garlic to taste
4. 1 tsp. toasted sesame oil for stir frying
5. Serve with 1 cup cooked brown rice or quinoa

Lunch Mixed Salad

How to make

1. Salad dressing: Use 1 tbs. of olive oil plus any vinegar that appeals to you.
2. Unlimited greens and other low-starch veggies from the Unlimited Foods list
3. ½ cup canned kidney or garbanzo beans

Chapter 9

These Food Are Not Limited In The Adrenal Reset Diet

- Alfalfa sprouts
- Artichokes
- Asparagus
- Baby corn
- Bamboo shoots
- Bean sprouts
- Bok Choy
- Broccoli
- Brussels sprouts
- Cabbage
- Carrots
- Cauliflower
- Celery
- Collard greens
- Cucumbers
- Daikon
- Eggplant
- Fennel
- Garlic
- Ginger
- Green beans
- Green onions
- Jicama

- Kohlrabi
- Leeks
- Lemon juice
- Lime juice
- Mushrooms
- Okra
- Onions
- Red Pepper
- Green pepper
- Radishes
- Rutabaga
- Any type of green salad
- Snow peas
- Spinach
- Summer squash (zucchini)
- Sunflower sprouts
- Swiss chard
- Tomatoes
- Tomatillos
- Turnip greens
- Water chestnuts
- Winter squash (pumpkin)

CHAPTER 10

FRUIT

Your intake of fruit is recommended to be limited. Apart from the berries you use in smoothies, you should really only eat fruit less than four times per week. Your ideal choices here would be one medium apple, one pear or a cup of melon cubes.

Fruit contains sugar in different forms, and so is not recommended on this diet. After you have used the Adrenal Reset Diet for a while, and notice a positive difference, then you may begin to reintroduce fruits to the diet slowly.

CHAPTER 11

Qigong for Adrenal Reset –

What Doctors & Dietitians Wont Teach You...

"Inner" Healing

Here in this part of the manual, we are going to present you a crucial aspect of healing. Title of the chapter is NOT the trick meant to grab you attention – it is real, more real than most people can imagine. Without touching ideas of those conspiracy theories and New World Order, we just have to conclude that most people today live in absurd and tragic situation. Here is why: There are simple yet effective methods for different health issues and conditions out there, but those are not available for most in need. That knowledge nowadays isn't easily reachable. With the power of Internet, this gets better and yet...

It's shocking to me (and probably most of you) to see how many people are totally misguided by false claims about getting fit and being healthy. You probably know already that powerful industrial lobbies own most of the media, pharmaceutical industry and sports nutrition market for example. In that way, they massively market and sell huge amount of vitamins, proteins, powders, drugs and pills under different labels.

All the misguided messages and avalanche of pharmaceutical and wellness/fitness marketing could get summed up in one sentence:

"Fitness and health comes from and it depends on outside factors."

Wrong, Wrong, WRONG! ... + verydangerous for everyone who believes in those claims.

You see, I don't mind that industry lobby magnates get richer and richer, if that's what they want to do. But it saddens me is to see an endless wave of illusion sold successfully to people. Believe me when I say...

...Most of today's approaches to healing, exercise and fitness are not at all healthy!

Why?

In short, the modern approaches and most of the medicine experts are aimed at the external aspects of the body ... cardiovascular system muscles, external symptoms of a disease etc.

What is wrong with that?

Well, a few things for starters. Our good health doesn't JUST depend on the heart, the muscles and the lungs. The healthy functioning of all organs in the body (kidneys, gall bladder, bladder, spleen, long & short intestine, etc.) directly provides us with good fitness level and health. NO health there = NO health at all! That means low energy, and a constant struggle with health. That is no way to achieve any decent fitness level, especially not in the long run.

In relation to that, (any type of) adrenal fatigue is very hard or nearly impossible to overcome without proper cure for the energy flow within the body and between the internal organs. Another way of showing this principle is through the ancient practice of Chi Kung. What we will offer to all of you is the quick way to solve this problem. Off course, video isn't most complete way to learn about the profound practice of Qigong and for that reason we are offering you here a brief overview and on the end of this chapter you will be instructed about how to get the Video. Exercises shown and explained in detail within Sifu Lee's Total Chi

<u>Fitness</u>book and we simply do not have time to do that here. What is important for you to know is that these simple stretching movements are aimed at reviving and maintaining a strong energy flow throughout our gross and subtle body.

Once healthy functioning of the internal organs has been achieved (supported by a lot of Chi and blood flow), we can start enjoying the benefits of total health and fitness in all eleven of our systems: cardiovascular, digestive, endocrine, lymphatic, immune, muscular, nervous, reproductive, respiratory, skeletal, and urinary. Now, I am sure you got interested, right?

Without having a healthy body on the inside, what is the point of talking about health, fitness, wellness and enjoying life? I hope you are with us on this. If you are and these words mean something to you, we know you will enjoy this book.

Proof is in the Pudding

Real value is not hidden in what someone says or writes. It is all about (and always was) the *practical benefits and results we actually get*. In our experience, the reality of life today demands an approach with as much practicality and efficiency as possible. Next to the previously explained differences, efficiency is the most prominent quality of Chi-Fitness exercises. In the same way as when Sifu is teaching a seminar or a private class, in this book I focus on practicality and efficiency inside of a process. You will be provided with a tool that you can use efficiently any time you want. If you do use it, you will be able to generate the same results as thousands of other practitioners – almost without being able to help it. The system is simple yet powerful, and people who use it start feeling the change in a fairly short time period. We <u>can</u> promise you that!

It is NOT only for the health problems and conditions connected with adrenal fatigue. Please check out the list bellow. These are main health issues that are treated and healed successfully with these simple exercises. By making your life Qi energy flow better trough out your body, limbs and organs you will influence many health disorders and conditions, just like was being done for thousands of years:

- Lack of energy
- Headache
- Difficulties in maintaining focus
- Feelings of physical weakness
- Mental weakness
- Need to boost your energy level
- Need to boost Sport performance
- Need to boost working performance
- Desire to boost weight loss results
- Need to improve detoxing results
- Suffering from chronic pain
- Allergies (including Gluten Intolerance)
- Difficulty enjoying life without painkillers and/or medication
- High or low blood pressure issues

- Suffering from a digestion disorders
- Need to accelerate healing from illness or surgery
- Desire to prevent the chronic "I am sick and tired" feeling
- Need to boost your libido and sex drive;

Now, everyone who had read my 5-Minute Chi Boost program will recognize this list of benefits. All are listed there as well. So, what is the difference between these two programs and why is that important for us?

In order to explain this in detail I need more space and therefore I'll do it right below.

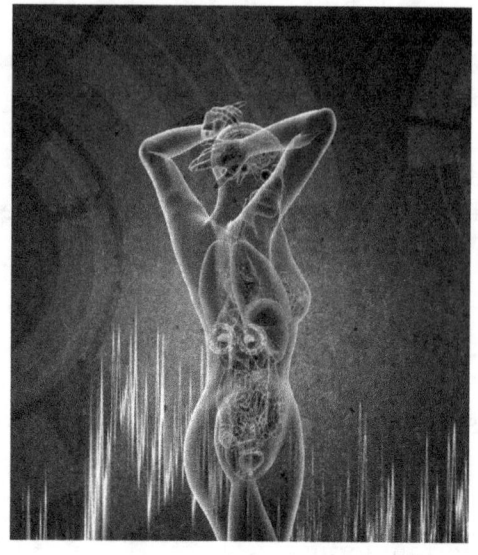

"5-Minute Boost" – "Total Chi Fitness": Difference

Here is the short answer: these are two separate programs. Both work well and help people. Like the content of a good electric razor, this is a total package meant for consistent home use, and the other is the smaller unit meant for traveling. Both are of superb quality, but one gets more done while the smaller one is easier to carry but must be used more frequently. Women might better understand example of pre-packaged hair dye; it works well to touch up color points, but getting a hair dye job done at a real salon will last for weeks longer.

The methods described in my first book, 5-Minute Chi Boost, are very effective, but you don't have to read them to benefit from this set of Qigong exercises.

Naturally, the acupressure techniques in 5-Minute Chi Boost are not the only healing exercises I teach. The reason for that is actually simple to understand. 5-Minute Chi Boost is a program that does exactly what it promises: boosts your Chi in matter of a few hours or days. Anyone who needs boost of energy and quick help will appreciate these methods. If you do like 5-Minute Chi Boost or similar acupressure routine, do it! There is nothing wrong in that – you will accelerate your energy cycles and quality of your life energy will increase.

Yet, in order to really start working on deep causes behind the Adrenal fatigue and the blockages that are causing so many (too many) health disorders, one needs more – the powerful meridian stretching routine. From there, the energy level of a busy practitioner only continues to increase. My first Kindle bestseller 5-Minute Chi Boostwas needed in order to offer the shortest and most practical Qi boosting program, so that people could generate the results really fast. If this is enough for you , great.

However, most people with Gluten intolerance troubles simply need to go deeper, with more profound practice. For that reason I recommend you to start with the Total Chi Fitness routine right away.

It is really interesting to read emails I get from people who take my books and use them in day-to-day life. The messages I get from those readers are very similar to those I've received over the last two and half decades of teaching. I'm very happy to read all reactions from people that read my book's on Amazon Kindle. Many readers give the identical feedback of the attendees at my 5-Minute Chi Boost seminar, after practicing the simple system for a while.

For example:

> "... I like the 5-Minute Chi Boost program. I get (such and such) benefit) when I do it. However, when I forget to do my 'cycle', my problems seems to reappear. Is there anything that has a longer lasting effect?

- *"I feel much better but I want more. My health problems seem to be deep-rooted can you show us something 'stronger'?"*

- *"In your book and in your email you are talking about assistance that is stronger and can help us even more. Where I can read more about that?"*

People ask this question in various

ways, conditioned by a range of circumstances in life. A few years back, I received an 18-page letter that essentially elaborated on only one of these questions. My answer always has been and still is the same.

My answer is "Yes", but you have to use common sense. No one can expect an instant 'magical' solution for a problem or a set of problems that have bothered you for several years or even decades. In the same way as I teach my students, I invite you to further expand the power and potency of the traditional art of Chi Kung. This book outlines complete Chi Kung exercises that have helped people for thousands of years – no question about that. They will also help you if you do them correctly. The learning curve is short, normally one or two weeks. However, you will need to set aside more time for doing them – not just five – ten minutes. Not to worry, it doesn't take a lot more time! Once learned, you can complete one Total Chi Fitness exercise set in about 15 to 20 minutes, and there is no need to repeat the cycle more than once. However, since autoimmune disorder such Celiac disease and gluten intolerance requires serious attention, you will need to be consistent in your practicing.

As you can see in Video that you receive with our book, the Total Chi Fitness program is fairly simple to perform and easy to learn. This routine influences each and every energy channel of the body, and can generate results that the 5-Minute Chi Boost program can't really offer to most practitioners and or most of the time. The main differences or additional benefits of Total Chi Fitness exercises are:

-Direct and stronger impact on root cause of health problems

-Higher strength for disease prevention

-Longer lasting effects on subtle and physical body

Simply speaking, these Total Chi Fitness Exercises are more profound and have longer lasting effects than anything else you may start practicing. The simple methods rely on stimulating pressure points and particularly generating a strong flow of life energy. Total Chi Fitness does the same, but by treating all meridians and pressure points on the body = full body. Compering these 2 approaches, one isn't better than the other – they are simply two programs with the same goals but a different approach.

Both can help you and both can heal you. If you have more health problems or if you are serious about preventing weakness, disease, lack of focus, tiredness, headaches (or the other symptoms listed above), I definitely recommend that you learn and start applying this program. If you only need a quick energy boost, just stick to methods described in the previously described book.

Powerful Qigong Routine Video

If you are not online right now while reading this book, you can always visit this link later. Please be advised, there is a necessary procedure, demanded due to anti spam rules and regulations.

1) First visit the link http://eepurl.com/6JUtPand subscribe to our list.
2) Confirm your email address
3) Please allow up to 1hfor system to register you. In maximum 1h time, you will be getting email with the link to the Total Chi Fitness Video.
4) If you do not see the Video after 1h, please check all the inboxes, spam filters etc. That usually solves a problem

Thank you.

More from the Authors:

QUICK GUIDE to VEGAN DIET & LIFESTYLE - PRACTICAL MANUAL THAT WILL ASSIST YOUR 'GOING & STAYING VEGAN

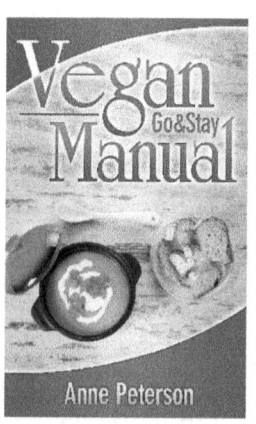

Shop on Amazon

(You DON'T necessarily need a Kindle reader device in order use this book. It's available for immediate reading with your Amazon virtual cloud reader).

Author who surprised readership with Golfing guide for the beginners 'Lifesaving' ABC Golf Instruction is coming with even bigger surprise. Switching to Vegan diet almost three decades ago, Mrs. Peterson grow more and more passionate about Vegan lifestyle, promoting it and assisting others in various matters connected to Vegan diet and lifestyle. Anne has managed to channel three decades of experience in this short, practical and easy to use form. This manual is filled with great looking photographs that add to smooth mood of this manual.

WARNING: THIS is NOT a cookbook - if you are looking for a collection of recipes and nothing else, you probably do not want this book. HOWEVER - VEGAN (Go & Stay) Manual will definitely enthuse your (Vegan cooking) creativity and ideas plus it will do for you so much more. Offering 'down to earth' guidelines, practical information and advice focused on health and well-being, Anne Peterson is avoiding all fluff, philosophical approaches and theories (that we normally find in most of the Vegan books not based on recipes). No one has to be worried about the title - this work in fact is a Manual. VEGAN (Go & Stay) Manual is not going to help only those man ans women who consider switching to Veganism but even to those that are already familiar with theory and practice of Vegan way of living.

In essence, what you see in front of you is quite unique, short yet very useful peace of information.

Make practical use of well-known wisdom lines such as 'KNOWLEDGE is the POWER'. HEALTHY VEGAN = HAPPY VEGAN – link to book

SIMPLE and DETAILED BEGGINERS GUIDE TO THE WORLD OF GOLF

That will save YOUR TIME & MONEY

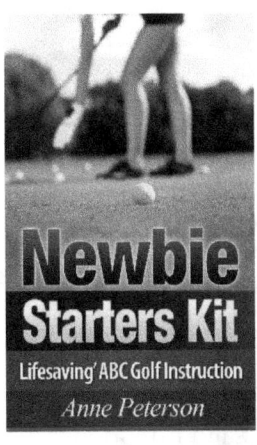

*Shop on Amazon**Anyone new (or not too experienced) to a game of Golf will definitely benefit from this guide immensely. You can start reading this book on Kindle device or computer right away.*

Unlike most Golf books we see around today, this guide is not presenting any sort of advanced knowledge, 'cool strategies, tactics and secrets'. Other books force a reader to turn in to 'more that he / she desires to be' – simple Golf lover and player for fun and enjoyment. Nothing like that you will find here. WHY? Well, nothing that is of sound quality, nothing really great or powerful in this world exists that without very firm and solid ground principles and basic knowledge. This really is a Newbie Starter Kit – simple yet fundamental for (any) Golfer.

I think you will agree with explanation how this book can boost up your Golfing carrier + safe you solid amounts of time and money. Here is just a thought: most people (not only newbies) fall pray to "ego trip" mind trick, mostly due to felling a social pressure. They start to artificially rush up the things in order to create illusion of "fast advancement" and in that way, many man and women miss to understand important aspects and gain basic understandings important for anyone who plays Golf. No amount of expensive special clothing and Golf gear can make you play better and no variety of cool tricks you learn from a book will help you either without having firm and solid BASIC UNDESRTANDING. So, I am not saying there is anything wrong with expensive gear and Golf clothes – I LOVE enjoying in those, as well. Out on the course, peace of mind is giving you more than all those things. In any case, If you consider yourself a beginner, nothing will help you more that simple and clear explanation of (practically) everything you need to know about and start your Golfing adventure.

SAFE YOUR TIME AND MONEY, KICKSTART YOU'RE GOLFING EXPERIENCE RIGHT NOW!

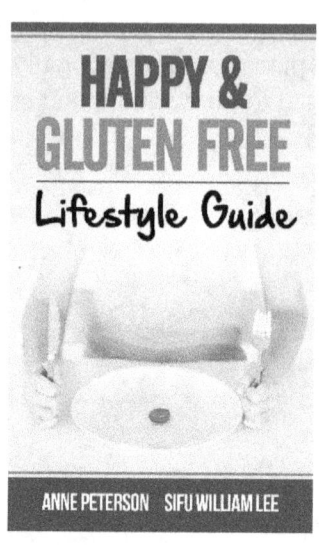

SIMPLE, PRACTI CAL Guide for Living a Happy GLUTEN FREE Lifestyle. This Book & Video Guide is Modern Approach Combined with EFFECTIVE Ancient Chinese Qigong Solution for Gluten Intolerance that will HELP you from Inside Out!

This practical guide contains probably most unique approach to Gluten intolerance lifestyle you can see around, due to very special co-authorship. Sifu William Lee's bestselling Amazon titles are assisting and healing thousands of people – this book will do the same. Anne Peterson on another hand, has the biggest qualification ever – being a mother of two children with developed gluten intolerance combined with her expertise in sector of Vegan and health food diet, makes her a 'real life' expert on the topics. Being a combined effort, this book is NOT meant for people looking after theory or statistics. It is loaded with very practical and effective solutions, information and tips - this book is created out from a need. COMBINED EFFORT: Having two children with developed gluten intolerance had forced Anne Peterson and her family to path of many tribulations - experimenting and searching out the best ways to live on a gluten free diet has became Ann's 'life mission'. As a passionate protagonist of healthy life and healthy (vegan) diet, in that effort, she probably had great advantage, if compared to someone without that experience. Nevertheless, new horizon's of living with and healing gluten intolerance opened as soon she came in contact with Sifu William Lee's books and teachings. HEALING from INSIDE OUT: Most people still consider the practices of Traditional

Chinese Medicine (TCM) complicated. But, if you take a look on any of the books written by Sifu Lee, you will realize very different truth. While Anne Peterson contributes here with amazingly simple approach to gluten free life, Sifu Lee is going to surprise most probably most of the readers here by his contribution. Here is why; most people that suffer from Gluten intolerance or Celiac disease do not even dream about possibility of becoming healed and yet, TCM presents several disciplines with potency to neutralize these health disorder. In this book, Sifu explains the basic facts and provided you with practical way to learn a Qiqong meridian stretching routine trough a simple Video presentation.

Regardless of who you are, if you are Gluten Intolerant (or you suspect that you may be), you need this guide. Anyone with open mind will be able to use this guide and benefit immensely from the tips, information, guidelines and practices presented within.

COMPLETE Guide for LIVING HAPPY GLUTEN FREE Life and HEALING From Gluten Intolerance!

Next Steps

Please, write us an honest review about the book – we truly value your opinion and thoughts and we will incorporate them into next book, which is already being prepared.

Leave your review of my book here: Here or simply On the **Kindle Page**

THANK YOU!

Sifu William Lee

<u>Amazon author Page</u>

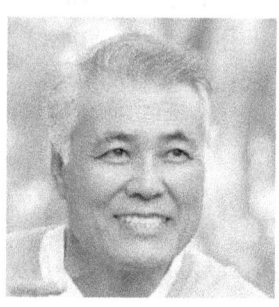

From early childhood on, I worked hard just to get food and water - times were extremely hard in Zhengzhou, China. When I was 5 years old, my mother had to leave my three sisters and me in order to survive. Though it seems like a terrible beginning, we all lived through it and gained great life experience. The will of providence brought me to work as a servant in the house of the great master, SifuQian Bo-Wan. His Kung Fu school became my home and shelter. At the age of 8, my passion for martial arts was recognized and I began learning personally from the great Bo-Wan.

I was trained in various methods: Wing Chun, Shao Lin Guan, Tai Chi Guan, Xing Xi Guam. I studied Chi Kung with my master and Buddhist monks. Just before my Sifu left this world, he told me: "Xi (his name for me), you have to go and spread this knowledge. You can do much more then I ever could, you will see." I felt humbled and obligated to carry out his wishes.

After finishing my studies of traditional Chinese medicine with Dr. Le Cai, I moved to the Western world. I have to admit, I never understood what my Sifu meant by 'you can do much more'. He did not say 'better', but more. I spent the last 30 years in teaching martial arts, Chi Kung, and related disciplines, but just recently I understood why he used the term 'much more'.

It was not because of anything in me. It is because of the Internet and modern technology that I really am able to fully fulfill his instructions. I am more than grateful to all my students and readers who help me, and continue reading and using my books. Thank you from the bottom of my heart, and God bless you.

DISCLAIMER

I am not a dietician, nor am I a doctor. I do not specialize in adrenal disorders. This eBook is not intended to take the place of your doctor's advice and treatment, but rather to help them work better. My idea for writing this book is to give you a better understanding of why you may need an Adrenal Reset Diet and to allow you to see there may be other reasons for why you cannot lose weight when you use the obvious ways of rearranging your diet and exercise.

The Adrenal Reset Diet may not be for everybody, which is why it is so important to consult your health professional or doctor before you undertake it. Long term medications, diet restrictions, allergies all are reasons you may not be able to take part fully in this diet. Although you must heed these restrictions, there is no reason why you cannot adopt moderations of the diet with your doctor's advice.

Resetting your Adrenal Glands can bring you improved health and energy as well as helping you to lose stubborn fat and improving the functions of many of your organs.

It should however be undertaken responsibly and with your doctor's permission.